INTERMITTENT FASTING FOR WOMEN

The Ultimate Guide To 90 Clean Eating Recipes To Boost Energy, Loss Weight, Eat Healthy, Delay Aging and Improve Hormonal Health

Sabestian Gastronomer

Copyright © 2023 by Sabestian Gastronomer

All Right Reserved

Any unauthorized use of any content or materials on this website is strictly prohibited and may violate copyright laws, trademark laws, laws of privacy and publicity, and other applicable regulations and statutes.

TABLE OF CONTENT

INTRODUCTION

The age of 50 marks a significant milestone in a woman's life, often accompanied by changes in metabolism, hormonal fluctuations, and unique health considerations. It is crucial for women in this age group to adopt a well-rounded approach to nutrition that supports their overall well-being. Intermittent fasting, a dietary practice that involves alternating periods of fasting and eating, has emerged as a popular and effective strategy for weight management, improved health, and increased longevity. Recognizing the specific needs of women over 50, a dedicated cookbook for intermittent fasting tailored to their requirements can be an invaluable resource.

The Intermittent Fasting for Women Over 50 Cookbook offers a comprehensive and practical guide to help women navigate the world of intermittent fasting while focusing on their nutritional needs and goals. This cookbook is designed to address the unique challenges faced by women in this age group, providing delicious and nutritious recipes that support their well-being and promote healthy aging.

Inside this cookbook, you will find a diverse range of recipes specifically curated to suit the intermittent fasting lifestyle of women over 50. From balanced and satisfying meals to nutrient-dense snacks and delightful desserts, each recipe is carefully crafted to provide the necessary nourishment while considering the potential health concerns and dietary preferences of this age group.

In addition to the mouthwatering recipes, this cookbook also includes valuable tips, guidance, and meal planning suggestions to help women over 50 successfully incorporate intermittent fasting into their lives. Whether you are new to intermittent fasting or looking to enhance your existing fasting routine, this cookbook serves as a trusted companion to support your journey towards optimal health and wellness.

With the Intermittent Fasting for Women Over 50 Cookbook, embrace the power of nutrition and intermittent fasting to unlock a healthier, more vibrant, and fulfilling life.

Meal Plan Guidelines:

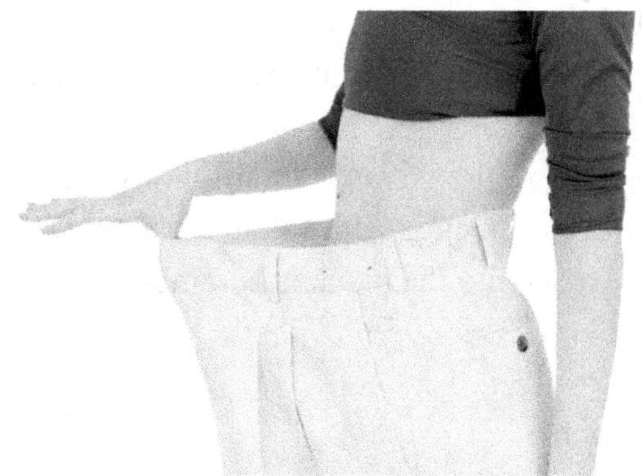

<u>Lose Weight Within 30 Days With This Meal Plan</u>

- 16:8 Method: Fasting for 16 hours and having an 8-hour eating window.
- Drink a lot of water all day long.
- Focus on whole, nutrient-dense foods.
- Adjust portion sizes based on your individual needs.

Day 1:

Meal 1 (Breakfast):
- Scrambled Eggs with Spinach and Mushrooms
Ingredients:
  - 2 eggs

- Handful of spinach
- 4-5 mushrooms, sliced
- Salt and pepper to taste

Preparation:

1. Heat a non-stick pan and sauté mushrooms until golden.

2. Once added, boil the spinach until it has wilted.

3. In a bowl, whisk eggs with salt and pepper.

4. Pour the eggs into the pan and scramble until cooked.

5. Serve hot.

Meal 2 (Lunch):

- Grilled Chicken Salad

Ingredients:

- 4 oz grilled chicken breast, sliced
- Mixed salad greens
- Cucumber, sliced
- Cherry tomatoes, halved
- Olive oil and vinegar dressing

Preparation:

1. Toss salad greens, cucumber, and cherry tomatoes in a bowl.

2. Add grilled chicken slices on top.

3. Drizzle with olive oil and vinegar dressing.

Meal 3 (Dinner):

- Baked Salmon with Roasted Vegetables

Ingredients:

- 4 oz salmon filet

- Various veggies, such as bell peppers, broccoli, and carrots

- Olive oil

- To season, use salt, pepper, and herbs.

Preparation:

1. Set the oven's temperature to 400°F (200°C).

2. Place salmon on a baking sheet lined with parchment paper.

3. Toss the vegetables with olive oil, salt, pepper, and herbs.

4. Around the salmon, arrange the vegetables.

5. Bake for 15 to 20 minutes, or until the veggies are soft and the salmon is cooked through.

Day 2:

Meal 1 (Breakfast):
- Greek Yogurt Parfait
Ingredients:

- 1 cup Greek yogurt

- Mixed berries (e.g., blueberries, strawberries)

- Chia seeds

- Nuts (e.g., almonds, walnuts)

Preparation:

1. In a glass or bowl, layer Greek yogurt, mixed berries, chia seeds, and nuts.

2. Repeat the layers as desired.

3. Serve chilled.

Meal 2 (Lunch):
- Black beans, Avocado, and Quinoa salad
Ingredients:
  - 1/2 cup cooked quinoa
  - 1/4 cup washed and drained black beans
  - 1/2 avocado, diced
  - Cherry tomatoes, halved
  - Fresh cilantro, chopped
  - Lime juice
  - Salt and pepper to taste
Preparation:
   1. In a bowl, combine cooked quinoa, black beans, avocado, cherry tomatoes, and cilantro.
   2. Squeeze lime juice over the salad and season with salt and pepper.
   3. Toss gently to mix well.

Meal 3 (Dinner):
- Grilled Turkey Breast with Steamed Vegetables
Ingredients:
  - 4 oz turkey breast
   - Assorted vegetables (e.g., broccoli, cauliflower, zucchini)
  - Garlic powder, paprika, and dried herbs for seasoning
Preparation:

1. Season the turkey breast with garlic powder, paprika, and dried herbs.

2. Cook the turkey completely on the grill.

3. Steam the vegetables until tender.

4. Serve the grilled turkey breast with steamed vegetables.

Day 3:

Meal 1 (Breakfast):
- Veggie Omelette
Ingredients:
- 2 eggs
- Bell peppers, diced
- Red onion, thinly sliced
- Spinach leaves
- Feta cheese, crumbled
- Salt and pepper to taste

Preparation:
1. Whisk eggs with salt and pepper in a bowl.

2. Heat a non-stick pan and sauté bell peppers and red onion until softened.

3. Add spinach leaves and cook until wilted.

4. Pour the eggs into the pan and cook until set.

5. Sprinkle feta cheese on top and fold the omelet.

6. Cook for another minute and serve hot.

Meal 2 (Lunch):
- Chickpea Salad
Ingredients:
  - 1 cup canned chickpeas, drained and rinsed
  - Cucumber, diced
  - Cherry tomatoes, halved
  - Red onion, thinly sliced
  - Kalamata olives
  - Feta cheese, crumbled
  - Lemon juice and olive oil dressing
Preparation:
  1. In a bowl, combine chickpeas, cucumber, cherry tomatoes, red onion, olives, and feta cheese.
  2. Drizzle with lemon juice and olive oil dressing.
  3. Toss gently to mix well.

Meal 3 (Dinner):
- Baked Cod with Roasted Asparagus
Ingredients:
  - 4 oz cod filet
  - Asparagus spears
  - Lemon slices
  - Garlic, minced
  - Olive oil
  - Salt and pepper to taste
Preparation:

1. Set the oven's temperature to 400°F (200°C).

2. Place cod filet on a baking sheet lined with parchment paper.

3. Drizzle with olive oil, sprinkle minced garlic, salt, and pepper.

4. Lemon slices should be placed on top of the fish.

5. Place asparagus spears on another baking sheet, drizzle with olive oil, salt, and pepper.

6. Bake both the cod and asparagus for 12-15 minutes or until the fish is cooked and the asparagus is tender.

Day 4:

Meal 1 (Breakfast):
- Overnight Chia Pudding
Ingredients:
- 2 tbsp chia seeds
- 1 cup almond milk (unsweetened)
- Mixed berries
- Unsweetened shredded coconut (optional)

Preparation:

1. In a jar or container, combine chia seeds and almond milk.

2. Stir well, then refrigerate overnight.

3. In the morning, top with mixed berries and shredded coconut.

Meal 2 (Lunch):
- Spinach Salad with Grilled Shrimp
Ingredients:
  - Handful of spinach leaves
  - Grilled shrimp
  - Cherry tomatoes, halved
  - Red bell pepper, sliced
  - Cucumber, sliced
  - Olive oil and balsamic vinegar dressing
Preparation:
  1. Toss spinach leaves, grilled shrimp, cherry tomatoes, red bell pepper, and cucumber in a bowl.
  2. Drizzle with balsamic vinegar and olive oil dressing.
  3. Toss gently to mix well.

Meal 3 (Dinner):
- Braised Brussels sprouts and baked chicken thighs
Ingredients:
  - 2 chicken thighs
  - Brussels sprouts
  - Garlic powder, paprika, and dried herbs for seasoning
  - Olive oil
  - Salt and pepper to taste
Preparation:
  1. Set the oven at 425°F (220°C).
  2. Season chicken thighs with garlic powder, paprika, dried herbs, salt, and pepper.

3. Place chicken thighs on a baking sheet lined with parchment paper.

4. Toss Brussels sprouts with olive oil, salt, and pepper.

5. Arrange Brussels sprouts around the chicken.

6. Bake for 25-30 minutes or until the chicken is cooked through and the Brussels sprouts are crispy.

Day 5:

Meal 1 (Breakfast):
- Vegetable Frittata
Ingredients:
- 2 eggs
- Zucchini, sliced
- Red bell pepper, diced
- Onion, diced
- Cherry tomatoes, halved
- Fresh basil, chopped
- Salt and pepper to taste

Preparation:
1. Set the oven at 375°F (190°C).

2. Whisk eggs with salt and pepper,in a bowl

3. Heat an oven-safe skillet and sauté zucchini, red bell pepper, and onion until softened.

4. Add cherry tomatoes and fresh basil, cook for another minute.

5. Pour the whisked eggs over the vegetables.

6. Transfer the skillet to the oven and bake for 12-15 minutes or until the frittata is set.

7. Slice and serve.

Meal 2 (Lunch):
- Lentil Soup
Ingredients:
 - 1 cup cooked lentils
 - Carrot, diced
 - Celery, diced
 - Onion, diced
 - Garlic, minced
 - Vegetable broth
 - Cumin, paprika, and dried herbs for seasoning
 - Salt and pepper to taste

Preparation:
1. In a pot, sauté carrot, celery, onion, and garlic until softened.

2. Add cooked lentils and vegetable broth.

3. Season with cumin, paprika, dried herbs, salt, and pepper.

4. Simmer for 15-20 minutes.

5. Adjust the seasoning if needed.

6. Serve hot.

Meal 3 (Dinner):
- Baked Tofu with Stir-Fried Vegetables
Ingredients:
  - 4 oz firm tofu, cubed
  - Assorted stir-fry vegetables (e.g., bell peppers, snap peas, carrots, broccoli)
  - Soy sauce
  - Sesame oil
  - Ginger, minced
  - Garlic, minced
  - Salt and pepper to taste
Preparation:
  1. Set the oven at 400°F (200°C).
  2. Place tofu cubes on a baking sheet lined with parchment paper.
  3. Drizzle with soy sauce, sesame oil, ginger, garlic, salt, and pepper.
  4. Bake for 20-25 minutes or until the tofu is golden and crispy.
  5. Meanwhile, stir-fry the vegetables in a pan with a little sesame oil until tender.
  6. Serve the baked tofu with stir-fried vegetables.

Day 6:

Meal 1 (Breakfast):
- Almond Butter Banana Smoothie
Ingredients:
  - 1 ripe banana
  - 2 tbsp almond butter
  - 1 cup almond milk (unsweetened)
  - 1 tsp honey (optional for added sweetness)
Preparation:
   1. In a blender, combine the banana, almond butter, almond milk, and honey.
   2. Blend until smooth and creamy.
   3. Place in a glass and sip.

Meal 2 (Lunch):
- Caprese Salad
Ingredients:
  - Fresh mozzarella cheese, sliced
  - Tomato, sliced
  - Fresh basil leaves
  - Balsamic glaze
  - Extra-virgin olive oil
  - Salt and pepper to taste
Preparation:
   1. Arrange the mozzarella cheese slices and tomato slices on a plate.
   2. Top with fresh basil leaves.

3. Olive oil and balsamic glaze should be drizzled.

4. Season with salt and pepper.

5. Serve at room temperature.

Meal 3 (Dinner):
- Grilled Steak with Steamed Broccoli
Ingredients:

- 4 oz steak (your preferred cut)

- Broccoli florets

- Garlic powder, onion powder, and black pepper for seasoning

- Olive oil

- Salt to taste

Preparation:

1. Preheat the grill.

2. Season the steak with garlic powder, onion powder, black pepper, and salt.

3. To get the desired degree of doneness, grill the steak.

4. Meanwhile, steam the broccoli until tender.

5. Drizzle the steamed broccoli with olive oil and sprinkle it with salt.

6. Serve the grilled steak with steamed broccoli.

Day 7:

Meal 1 (Breakfast):
- Spinach and Mushroom Frittata
Ingredients:
  - 2 eggs
  - Handful of spinach leaves
  - 4-5 mushrooms, sliced
  - Onion, diced
  - Garlic, minced
  - Salt and pepper to taste

Preparation:
  1. Heat a non-stick pan and sauté the mushrooms, onion, and garlic until softened.
  2. Add the spinach leaves and cook until wilted.
  3. Whisk the eggs with salt and pepper in a bowl.
  4. Pour the whisked eggs into the pan and cook until set.
  5. Slice the frittata into wedges and serve.

Meal 2 (Lunch):
- Greek Salad with Grilled Chicken
Ingredients:
  - 4 oz grilled chicken breast, sliced
  - Mixed salad greens
  - Cucumber, diced
  - Cherry tomatoes, halved
  - Kalamata olives

- Feta cheese, crumbled
- Lemon juice and olive oil dressing

Preparation:

1. Toss the salad greens, cucumber, cherry tomatoes, olives, and feta cheese in a bowl.

2. Add the sliced grilled chicken on top.

3. Drizzle with lemon juice and olive oil dressing.

4. Toss gently to mix well.

Meal 3 (Dinner):
- Baked Halibut with Sautéed Spinach
Ingredients:

- 4 oz halibut filet
- Lemon juice
- Dried dill
- Olive oil
- Salt and pepper to taste
- Fresh spinach leaves
- Garlic, minced
- Red pepper flakes (optional)

Preparation:

1. Set the oven at 375°F (190°C).

2. On a baking sheet covered with parchment paper, put the halibut filet.

3. Drizzle with lemon juice, dried dill, olive oil, salt, and pepper.

4. Bake the fish for 12 to 15 minutes, or until it is thoroughly done.

5. Meanwhile, heat a pan with a little olive oil.

6. Sauté the garlic and red pepper flakes (if using) until fragrant.

7. Add the spinach leaves and cook until wilted.

8. Serve the baked halibut with sautéed spinach.

Day 8:

Meal 1 (Breakfast):
- Veggie Omelette
Ingredients:
- 2 eggs
- Bell peppers, diced
- Onion, diced
- Tomatoes, diced
- chopped fresh herbs (like parsley or basil)
- Salt and pepper to taste

Preparation:
1. Whisk the eggs with salt and pepper in a bowl

2. Heat a non-stick pan and sauté the bell peppers and onion until softened.

3. Add the tomatoes and fresh herbs, and cook for another minute.

4. Pour the whisked eggs into the pan and cook until set.

5. Fold the omelet and cook for an additional minute.

6. Slice and serve.

Meal 2 (Lunch):
- Quinoa and Vegetable Stir-Fry
Ingredients:
  - 1/2 cup cooked quinoa
  - Assorted stir-fry vegetables (e.g., broccoli, snap peas, carrots, bell peppers)
  - Garlic, minced
  - Soy sauce
  - Sesame oil
  - Salt and pepper to taste

Preparation:
  1. Heat a pan or wok with a little sesame oil.
  2. Sauté the garlic until fragrant.
  3. Add the stir-fry vegetables and cook until tender-crisp.
  4. Stir in the cooked quinoa and season with soy sauce, salt, and pepper.
  5. Stir-fry for another minute to combine the flavors.
  6. Serve hot.

Meal 3 (Dinner):
- Stuffed Bell Peppers
Ingredients:
  - Bell peppers
  - Lean ground turkey or chicken
  - Onion, diced
  - Garlic, minced

- Tomato sauce (sugar-free)
- Cooked quinoa
- chopped fresh herbs (like parsley or basil)
- Salt and pepper to taste

Preparation:

1. Set the oven at 375°F (190°C).

2. The bell peppers' tops should be cut off, and the seeds and membranes should be removed.

3. In a pan, cook the ground turkey or chicken with diced onion and minced garlic until browned.

4. Stir in the tomato sauce, cooked quinoa, fresh herbs, salt, and pepper.

5. Spoon the filling into the hollowed-out bell peppers.

6. Place the stuffed peppers in a baking dish and bake for 25-30 minutes or until the peppers are tender and the filling is cooked through.

Day 9:

Meal 1 (Breakfast):
- Berry and Nut Overnight Oats
Ingredients:
- 1/2 cup rolled oats
- 1/2 cup almond milk (unsweetened)
- Mixed berries (e.g., blueberries, raspberries)
- Chopped nuts (e.g., almonds, walnuts)
- Honey or maple syrup (optional for added sweetness)

Preparation:

1. In a jar or container, combine the rolled oats and almond milk.

2. Stir well, then refrigerate overnight.

3. In the morning, top with mixed berries and chopped nuts.

4. If desired, drizzle with honey or maple syrup.

Meal 2 (Lunch):
- Tuna Salad Lettuce Wraps
Ingredients:
- tuna in water-packed cans that has been drained
- Celery, diced
- Red onion, diced
- Dill pickles, diced
- Greek yogurt
- Dijon mustard
- Salt and pepper to taste
- the leaves of lettuce (such as romaine or butter lettuce).

Preparation:
1. In a bowl, combine the tuna, celery, red onion, dill pickles, Greek yogurt, Dijon mustard, salt, and pepper.

2. Mix well to combine.

3. Spoon the tuna salad onto the lettuce leaves and wrap them up.

4. Serve chilled.

Meal 3 (Dinner):
- Baked Chicken with Roasted Vegetables
Ingredients:
- 4 oz chicken breast
- Assorted vegetables (e.g., Brussels sprouts, carrots, sweet potatoes)
- Olive oil
- Garlic powder, paprika, and dried herbs for seasoning
- Salt and pepper to taste

Preparation:
1. Set the oven at 400°F (200°C).
2. Season the chicken breast with garlic powder, paprika, dried herbs, salt, and pepper.
3. Arrange the chicken breast on a parchment-lined baking pan.
4. Add salt, pepper, and olive oil to the vegetables.
5. Arrange the chicken with the vegetables.
6. Bake for 25-30 minutes or until the chicken is cooked through and the vegetables are tender.

Day 10:

Meal 1 (Breakfast):
- Veggie and Cheese Omelette
Ingredients:
- 2 eggs
- Bell peppers, diced
- Onion, diced

- Spinach leaves
- Cheddar or feta cheese that has been shredded
- Salt and pepper to taste

Preparation:

1. Whisk the eggs with salt and pepper in a bowl
2. Heat a non-stick pan and sauté the bell peppers and onion until softened.
3. Spinach leaves should be added and cooked until wilted.
4. Pour the whisked eggs into the pan and cook until set.
5. Sprinkle shredded cheese on one side of the omelet.
6. Fold the omelet in half to cover the cheese.
7. Cook for another minute to melt the cheese.
8. Slice and serve.

Meal 2 (Lunch):

- Mediterranean Salad with Grilled Shrimp

Ingredients:

- Grilled shrimp
- Mixed salad greens
- Cucumber, sliced
- Cherry tomatoes, halved
- Red onion, thinly sliced
- Kalamata olives
- Feta cheese, crumbled
- Lemon juice and olive oil dressing

Preparation:

1. Toss the salad greens, cucumber, cherry tomatoes, red onion, olives, and feta cheese in a bowl.

2. Add the grilled shrimp on top.

3. Drizzle with lemon juice and olive oil dressing.

4. Toss gently to mix well.

Meal 3 (Dinner):

- Quinoa-based baked cod dish with steamed vegetables

Ingredients:

- 4 oz cod filet

- Lemon juice

- Dried dill

- Olive oil

- Salt and pepper to taste

- 1/2 cup cooked quinoa

- Assorted steamed vegetables (e.g., broccoli, carrots, cauliflower)

Preparation:

1. Set the oven to 375°F (190°C).

2. The fish filet should be put on a baking pan covered with parchment paper.

3. Drizzle with lemon juice, dried dill, olive oil, salt, and pepper.

4. Bake the fish for 12 to 15 minutes, or until it is thoroughly done.

5. Meanwhile, prepare the quinoa according to package instructions.

6. Steam the vegetables until tender.

7. Serve the baked cod with quinoa and steamed vegetables.

Day 11:

Meal 1 (Breakfast):
- Greek Yogurt with Berries and Almonds
Ingredients:
- 1 cup Greek yogurt
- Mixed berries (e.g., blueberries, strawberries, raspberries)
- Almonds, sliced
- Honey (optional)
Preparation:
1. In a bowl, scoop the Greek yogurt.
2. Top with mixed berries and sliced almonds.
3. Drizzle with honey if desired.
4. Enjoy!

Meal 2 (Lunch):
- Chicken Caesar Salad
Ingredients:
- Grilled chicken breast, sliced
- Romaine lettuce, chopped
- Parmesan cheese, grated

- Whole wheat croutons
- Caesar dressing (look for a low-fat or homemade version)

Preparation:

1. In a large bowl, combine the romaine lettuce, grilled chicken breast, Parmesan cheese, and croutons.
2. Drizzle with Caesar dressing.
3. Toss gently to coat the ingredients.
4. Serve fresh.

Meal 3 (Dinner):

- Salmon baked with quinoa and asparagus steaming

Ingredients:

- 4 oz salmon filet
- Lemon juice
- Dried herbs (like thyme or dill)
- Olive oil
- Salt and pepper to taste
- 1/2 cup cooked quinoa
- Asparagus spears

Preparation:

1. Set the oven to 400°F (200°C).
2. Place the salmon filet on a baking sheet lined with parchment paper.
3. Squeeze lemon juice over the salmon.
4. Sprinkle dried herbs, salt, and pepper.
5. Drizzle with olive oil.

6. Bake for 12-15 minutes or until the salmon is cooked through.

7. Meanwhile, steam the asparagus until tender.

8. Serve the baked salmon with cooked quinoa and steamed asparagus.

Day 12:

Meal 1 (Breakfast):
- Vegetable and Cheese Frittata
Ingredients:
- 2 eggs
- Bell peppers, diced
- Onion, diced
- Spinach leaves
- Shredded cheese (such as cheddar or mozzarella)
- Salt and pepper to taste
Preparation:
1. Whisk the eggs with salt and pepper in a bowl
2. Heat a non-stick pan and sauté the bell peppers and onion until softened.
3. Once added, boil the spinach until it has wilted.
4. Pour the whisked eggs into the pan and cook until set.
5. Sprinkle shredded cheese on top.
6. Cook for another minute until the cheese melts.
7. Slice and serve.

Meal 2 (Lunch):
- Quinoa and Black Bean Salad
Ingredients:
- 1/2 cup cooked quinoa
- 1/2 cup canned black beans, drained and rinsed
- Cherry tomatoes, halved
- Red onion, diced
- Cucumber, diced
- Fresh cilantro, chopped
- Lime juice
- Olive oil
- Salt and pepper to taste

Preparation:
1. In a bowl, combine the cooked quinoa, black beans, cherry tomatoes, red onion, cucumber, and fresh cilantro.
2. Squeeze lime juice over the salad.
3. Drizzle with olive oil.
4. Season with salt and pepper.
5. Toss gently to mix well.

Meal 3 (Dinner):
- Grilled Chicken with Roasted Vegetables
Ingredients:
- 4 oz chicken breast
- Assorted vegetables (e.g., bell peppers, zucchini, eggplant)

- Olive oil
- Garlic powder, paprika, and dried herbs for seasoning
- Salt and pepper to taste
Preparation:
1. Preheat the grill.
2. Season the chicken breast with garlic powder, paprika, dried herbs, salt, and pepper.
3. Grill the chicken until cooked through.
4. Meanwhile, preheat the oven to 400°F (200°C).
5. Toss the vegetables with olive oil, salt, and pepper.
6. Spread the vegetables on a baking sheet and roast for 15-20 minutes or until tender.
7. Serve the grilled chicken with roasted vegetables.

Day 13:

Meal 1 (Breakfast):
- Spinach and Mushroom Omelette
Ingredients:
- 2 eggs
- Spinach leaves
- Mushrooms, sliced
- Onion, diced
- Garlic, minced
- Salt and pepper to taste
Preparation:
1. Whisk the eggs with salt and pepper in a bowl

2. Heat a non-stick pan and sauté the mushrooms, onion, and garlic until softened.

3. Once added, boil the spinach until it has wilted.

4. Pour the whisked eggs into the pan and cook until set.

5. Fold the omelet in half and cook for another minute.

6. Slice and serve.

Meal 2 (Lunch):
- Lentil Soup with Salad
Ingredients:
- 1 cup cooked lentils
- Carrot, diced
- Celery, diced
- Onion, diced
- Garlic, minced
- Vegetable broth
- Cumin, paprika, and dried herbs for seasoning
- Salt and pepper to taste
- Mixed salad greens
- Cherry tomatoes, halved
- Cucumber, sliced
- Balsamic vinegar and olive oil dressing
Preparation:
1. In a pot, sauté the carrot, celery, onion, and garlic until softened.

2. Add the cooked lentils and vegetable broth.

3. Season with cumin, paprika, dried herbs, salt, and pepper.

4. Simmer for 15-20 minutes.

5. Adjust the seasoning if needed.

6. Serve the lentil soup with a side salad of mixed greens, cherry tomatoes, and cucumber.

7. Drizzle with balsamic vinegar and olive oil dressing.

Meal 3 (Dinner):

- Baked Cod with Stir-Fried Vegetables

Ingredients:

- 4 oz cod filet

- Lemon juice

- Dried herbs (like rosemary or thyme)

- Olive oil

- Salt and pepper to taste

- Assorted stir-fry vegetables (e.g., broccoli, bell peppers, snow peas)

- Garlic, minced

- Soy sauce

- Sesame oil

Preparation:

1. Preheat the oven to 400°F (200°C).

2. On a baking sheet covered with parchment paper, put the cod filet.

3. Squeeze lemon juice over the fish.

4. Sprinkle dried herbs, salt, and pepper.

5. Drizzle with olive oil.

6. Bake for 12-15 minutes or until the fish is cooked through.

7. Meanwhile, heat a pan with a little sesame oil.

8. Sauté the minced garlic until fragrant.

9. Add the stir-fry vegetables and cook until tender-crisp.

10. Drizzle with soy sauce and toss to coat.

11. Serve the baked cod with stir-fried vegetables.

Day 14:

Meal 1 (Breakfast):
- Berry Protein Smoothie
Ingredients:
- 1 cup unsweetened almond milk
-1 scoop of the protein powder you choose
- Mixed berries (e.g., strawberries, blueberries, raspberries)
- 1 tbsp almond butter
- Ice cubes (optional)
Preparation:
1. In a blender, combine the almond milk, protein powder, mixed berries, almond butter, and ice cubes.

2. Blend until smooth and creamy.

3. Pour into a glass and enjoy.

Meal 2 (Lunch):
- Greek Salad Wrap
Ingredients:
- Whole wheat tortilla
- Mixed salad greens

- Cucumber, sliced
- Cherry tomatoes, halved
- Red onion, thinly sliced
- Kalamata olives
- Feta cheese, crumbled
- Greek yogurt
- Dried oregano

Preparation:

1. Lay the whole wheat tortilla flat.
2. Spread Greek yogurt on the tortilla.
3. Layer mixed salad greens, cucumber slices, cherry tomatoes, red onion, olives, and feta cheese.
4. Sprinkle dried oregano.
5. Roll the tortilla into a wrap.
6. Serve fresh or lightly toasted.

Meal 3 (Dinner):
- Baked Chicken Thighs with Quinoa and Steamed Broccoli

Ingredients:

- 2 chicken thighs
- Lemon juice
- Garlic powder, paprika, and dried herbs for seasoning
- Olive oil
- Salt and pepper to taste
- 1/2 cup cooked quinoa
- Broccoli florets

Preparation:

1. Preheat the oven to 425°F (220°C).
2. Season the chicken thighs with garlic powder, paprika, dried herbs, salt, and pepper.
3. Place the chicken thighs on a baking sheet lined with parchment paper.
4. Squeeze lemon juice over the chicken.
5. Drizzle with olive oil.
6. Bake for 25-30 minutes or until the chicken is cooked through and the skin is crispy.
7. Meanwhile, steam the broccoli florets until tender.
8. Serve the baked chicken thighs with cooked quinoa and steamed broccoli.

Day 15:

Meal 1 (Breakfast):
- Vegetable Omelet
Ingredients:
- 2 eggs
- Bell peppers, diced
- Onion, diced
- Spinach leaves
- Tomatoes, diced
- Salt and pepper to taste
- chopped fresh herbs (like parsley or basil)
Preparation:
1. Whisk the eggs with salt and pepper in a bowl

2. Heat a non-stick pan and sauté the bell peppers and onion until softened.

3. Once added, boil the spinach until it has wilted.

4. Add the tomatoes and fresh herbs, and cook for another minute.

5. Pour the whisked eggs into the pan and cook until set.

6. Fold the omelet in half and cook for an additional minute.

7. Slice and serve.

Meal 2 (Lunch):
- Quinoa and Chickpea Salad
Ingredients:
- 1/2 cup cooked quinoa
- 1/2 cup washed and drained canned chickpeas
- Cucumber, diced
- Cherry tomatoes, halved
- Red onion, thinly sliced
- Fresh parsley, chopped
- Lemon juice
- Olive oil
- Salt and pepper to taste
Preparation:
1. In a bowl, combine the cooked quinoa, chickpeas, cucumber, cherry tomatoes, red onion, and fresh parsley.

2. Squeeze lemon juice over the salad.

3. Drizzle with olive oil.

4. Season with salt and pepper.

5. Toss gently to mix well.

Meal 3 (Dinner):
- Grilled Salmon with Roasted Brussels Sprouts
Ingredients:
- 4 oz salmon filet
- Lemon juice
- Dried dill
- Olive oil
- Salt and pepper to taste
- Brussels sprouts
- Garlic powder
- Olive oil
- Salt and pepper to taste
Preparation:
1. Preheat the grill.
2. Season the salmon filet with lemon juice, dried dill, olive oil, salt, and pepper.
3. Grill the salmon until cooked through.
4. Meanwhile, preheat the oven to 400°F (200°C).
5. Toss the Brussels sprouts with garlic powder, olive oil, salt, and pepper.
6. Spread the Brussels sprouts on a baking sheet and roast for 20-25 minutes or until tender.
7. Serve the grilled salmon with roasted Brussels sprouts.

Day 16:

Meal 1 (Breakfast):
- Berry and Spinach Smoothie
Ingredients:
- 1 cup almond milk (unsweetened)
- Mixed berries (e.g., blueberries, strawberries, raspberries)
- Spinach leaves
- 1 tbsp almond butter
- Ice cubes (optional)
Preparation:
1. In a blender, combine the almond milk, mixed berries, spinach leaves, almond butter, and ice cubes.
2. Blend until smooth and creamy.
3. Pour into a glass and enjoy.

Meal 2 (Lunch):
- Greek Chicken Salad
Ingredients:
- Grilled chicken breast, sliced
- Mixed salad greens
- Cucumber, sliced
- Cherry tomatoes, halved
- Kalamata olives
- Feta cheese, crumbled
- Lemon juice and olive oil dressing
- Dried oregano

Preparation:

1. Toss the salad greens, cucumber, cherry tomatoes, Kalamata olives, and feta cheese in a bowl.

2. Add the sliced grilled chicken on top.

3. Drizzle with lemon juice and olive oil dressing.

4. Sprinkle dried oregano.

5. Toss gently to mix well.

Meal 3 (Dinner):
- Baked Chicken Breast with Steamed Vegetables
Ingredients:
- 4 oz chicken breast
- Lemon juice
- Garlic powder, paprika, and dried herbs for seasoning
- Olive oil
- Salt and pepper to taste
- Assorted steamed vegetables (e.g., broccoli, carrots, cauliflower)
Preparation:
1. Preheat the oven to 400°F (200°C).

2. Season the chicken breast with lemon juice, garlic powder, paprika, dried herbs, salt, and pepper.

3. Drizzle with olive oil.

4. Place the chicken breast on a baking sheet lined with parchment paper.

5. Bake the chicken for 20 to 25 minutes, or until cooked through.

6. Meanwhile, steam the vegetables until tender.

7. Serve the baked chicken breast with steamed vegetables.

Day 17:

Meal 1 (Breakfast):
- Vegetable Scramble
Ingredients:
- 2 eggs
- Bell peppers, diced
- Onion, diced
- Spinach leaves
- Tomatoes, diced
- Salt and pepper to taste
- Chopped fresh herbs (such as parsley or basil).
Preparation:
1. Whisk the eggs with salt and pepper in a bowl
2. Heat a non-stick pan and sauté the bell peppers and onion until softened.
3. Once added, boil the spinach until it has wilted.
4. Add the tomatoes and fresh herbs, and cook for another minute.
5. Pour the whisked eggs into the pan and scramble until cooked.
6. Serve hot.

Meal 2 (Lunch):
- Mediterranean Quinoa Bowl
Ingredients:
- 1/2 cup cooked quinoa
- Cucumber, diced
- Cherry tomatoes, halved
- Red onion, thinly sliced
- Kalamata olives
- Feta cheese, crumbled
- Fresh parsley, chopped
- Lemon juice
- Olive oil
- Salt and pepper to taste

Preparation:
1. In a bowl, combine the cooked quinoa, cucumber, cherry tomatoes, red onion, Kalamata olives, feta cheese, and fresh parsley.
2. Squeeze lemon juice over the quinoa bowl.
3. Drizzle with olive oil.
4. Season with salt and pepper.
5. Toss gently to mix well.

Meal 3 (Dinner):
- Quinoa and Roasted Asparagus with Baked Cod
Ingredients:
- 4 oz cod filet
- Lemon juice
- Dried herbs (such as Rosemary or thyme)

- Olive oil
- Salt and pepper to taste
- 1/2 cup cooked quinoa
- Asparagus spears
- Olive oil
- Garlic powder
- Salt and pepper to taste

Preparation:

1. Preheat the oven to 400°F (200°C).

2. On a baking sheet covered with parchment paper, put the cod filet.

3. Squeeze lemon juice over the fish.

4. Sprinkle dried herbs, salt, and pepper.

5. Drizzle with olive oil.

6. Bake for 12-15 minutes or until the fish is cooked through.

7. Meanwhile, preheat the oven to 425°F (220°C).

8. Toss the asparagus spears with olive oil, garlic powder, salt, and pepper.

9. Spread the asparagus on a baking sheet and roast for 12-15 minutes or until tender.

10. Serve the baked cod with cooked quinoa and roasted asparagus.

Day 18:

Meal 1 (Breakfast):
- Almond Butter Banana Toast
Ingredients:
- Whole wheat bread (toasted)
- Almond butter
- Ripe banana, sliced
- Chia seeds (optional)
Preparation:
1. Toast the whole wheat bread.
2. Spread almond butter on the toast.
3. Top with sliced banana.
4. Sprinkle chia seeds if desired.
5. Enjoy!

Meal 2 (Lunch):
- Lentil Soup with Side Salad
Ingredients:
- 1 cup cooked lentils
- Carrot, diced
- Celery, diced
- Onion, diced
- Garlic, minced
- Vegetable broth
- Cumin, paprika, and dried herbs for seasoning
- Salt and pepper to taste
- Mixed salad greens

- Cherry tomatoes, halved
- Cucumber, sliced
- Balsamic vinegar and olive oil dressing

Preparation:

1. In a pot, sauté the carrot, celery, onion, and garlic until softened.

2. Add the cooked lentils and vegetable broth.

3. Season with cumin, paprika, dried herbs, salt, and pepper.

4. Simmer for 15-20 minutes.

5. Adjust the seasoning if needed.

6. Serve the lentil soup with a side salad of mixed greens, cherry tomatoes, and cucumber.

7. Drizzle with balsamic vinegar and olive oil dressing.

Meal 3 (Dinner):
- Grilled Chicken with Stir-Fried Vegetables
Ingredients:
- 4 oz chicken breast
- Lemon juice
- Garlic powder, paprika, and dried herbs for seasoning
- Olive oil
- Salt and pepper to taste
- Assorted stir-fry vegetables (e.g., bell peppers, broccoli, snap peas)
- Garlic, minced
- Soy sauce
- Sesame oil

Preparation:

1. Preheat the grill.
2. Season the chicken breast with lemon juice, garlic powder, paprika, dried herbs, salt, and pepper.
3. Drizzle with olive oil.
4. Grill the chicken until cooked through.
5. Meanwhile, heat a pan with a little sesame oil.
6. Sauté the minced garlic until fragrant.
7. Add the stir-fry vegetables and cook until tender-crisp.
8. Drizzle with soy sauce and toss to coat.
9. Serve the grilled chicken with stir-fried vegetables.

Day 19:

Meal 1 (Breakfast):
- Vegetable and Cheese Frittata
Ingredients:
- 2 eggs
- Bell peppers, diced
- Onion, diced
- Spinach leaves
- Tomatoes, diced
- Salt and pepper to taste
- Chopped fresh herbs (such as parsley or basil).

Preparation:
1. Whisk the eggs with salt and pepper in a bowl
2. Heat a non-stick pan and sauté the bell peppers and onion until softened.

3. Once added, boil the spinach until it has wilted.

4. Add the tomatoes and fresh herbs, and cook for another minute.

5. Pour the whisked eggs into the pan and cook until set.

6. Fold the frittata in half and cook for an additional minute.

7. Slice and serve.

Meal 2 (Lunch):

- Chickpea Salad Wrap

Ingredients:

- Whole wheat tortilla

- Chickpeas, mashed or lightly mashed

- Red onion, diced

- Celery, diced

- Fresh parsley, chopped

- Greek yogurt or hummus

- Lemon juice

- Salt and pepper to taste

Preparation:

1. Lay the whole wheat tortilla flat.

2. Spread Greek yogurt or hummus on the tortilla.

3. Spread mashed chickpeas on top.

4. Add diced red onion, diced celery, and fresh parsley.

5. Squeeze lemon juice over the filling.

6. Season with salt and pepper.

7. Roll the tortilla into a wrap.

8. Serve fresh or lightly toasted.

Meal 3 (Dinner):
- Baked Salmon with Quinoa and Steamed Broccoli
Ingredients:
- 4 oz salmon filet
- Lemon juice
- Dried dill
- Olive oil
- Salt and pepper to taste
- 1/2 cup cooked quinoa
- Broccoli florets
Preparation:
1. Preheat the oven to 375°F (190°C).
2. Place the salmon filet on a baking sheet lined with parchment paper.
3. Squeeze lemon juice over the salmon.
4. Sprinkle dried dill, salt, and pepper.
5. Drizzle with olive oil.
6. Bake for 12-15 minutes or until the salmon is cooked through.
7. Meanwhile, steam the broccoli florets until tender.
8. Serve the baked salmon with cooked quinoa and steamed broccoli.

Day 20:

Meal 1 (Breakfast):
- **Mixed Berry Overnight Oats**
Ingredients:
- 1/2 cup rolled oats
- 1/2 cup almond milk (unsweetened)
- Mixed berries (e.g., blueberries, strawberries, raspberries)
- Chia seeds
- Maple syrup or Honey (optional for added sweetness)
Preparation:
1. In a jar or container, combine the rolled oats and almond milk.
2. Add mixed berries and chia seeds.
3. Stir well, then refrigerate overnight.
4. In the morning, give it a good stir.
5. If desired, drizzle with honey or maple syrup for added sweetness.
6. Enjoy it cold or heat it up in the microwave.

Meal 2 (Lunch):
- **Greek Salad with Grilled Shrimp**
Ingredients:
- Grilled shrimp
- Mixed salad greens
- Cucumber, sliced
- Cherry tomatoes, halved

- Red onion, thinly sliced
- Kalamata olives
- Feta cheese, crumbled
- Lemon juice and olive oil dressing
- Dried oregano

Preparation:

1. Toss the salad greens, cucumber, cherry tomatoes, red onion, Kalamata olives, and feta cheese in a bowl.
2. Add the grilled shrimp on top.
3. Drizzle with lemon juice and olive oil dressing.
4. Sprinkle dried oregano.
5. Toss gently to mix well.

Meal 3 (Dinner):
- Baked Chicken Thighs with Roasted Vegetables
Ingredients:
- 2 chicken thighs
- Assorted vegetables (e.g., bell peppers, zucchini, eggplant)
- Olive oil
- Garlic powder, paprika, and dried herbs for seasoning
- Salt and pepper to taste

Preparation:

1. Preheat the oven to 425°F (220°C).
2. Season the chicken thighs with garlic powder, paprika, dried herbs, salt, and pepper.
3. Place the chicken thighs on a baking sheet lined with parchment paper.

4. Drizzle with olive oil.

5. Toss the vegetables with olive oil, salt, and pepper.

6. Spread the vegetables around the chicken thighs.

7. Bake for 25-30 minutes or until the chicken is cooked through and the vegetables are tender.

Day 21:

Meal 1 (Breakfast):
- Veggie and Cheese Omelette
Ingredients:
- 2 eggs
- Bell peppers, diced
- Onion, diced
- Spinach leaves
- Shredded cheese (such as feta or cheddar)
- Salt and pepper to taste
Preparation:
1. Whisk the eggs with salt and pepper in a bowl

2. Heat a non-stick pan and sauté the bell peppers and onion until softened.

3. Once added, boil the spinach until it has wilted.

4. Pour the whisked eggs into the pan and cook until set.

5. Sprinkle shredded cheese on one side of the omelet.

6. Fold the omelet in half to cover the cheese.

7. Cook for another minute to melt the cheese.

8. Slice and serve.

Meal 2 (Lunch):
- Quinoa and Chickpea Salad
Ingredients:
- 1/2 cup cooked quinoa
- 1/2 cup washed and drained canned chickpeas
- Cucumber, diced
- Cherry tomatoes, halved
- Red onion, thinly sliced
- Fresh parsley, chopped
- Lemon juice and olive oil dressing
- Salt and pepper to taste

Preparation:
1. In a bowl, combine the cooked quinoa, chickpeas, cucumber, cherry tomatoes, red onion, and fresh parsley.
2. Drizzle with lemon juice and olive oil dressing.
3. Season with salt and pepper.
4. Toss gently to mix well.

Meal 3 (Dinner):
- Baked Salmon with Roasted Vegetables
Ingredients:
- 4 oz salmon filet
- Lemon juice
- Dried dill
- Olive oil
- Salt and pepper to taste
- Vegetables (e.g., broccoli, carrots, bell peppers) assorted

- Garlic powder
- Olive oil
- Salt and pepper to taste
Preparation:
1. Preheat the oven to 400°F (200°C).
2. Place the salmon filet on a baking sheet lined with parchment paper.
3. Squeeze lemon juice over the salmon.
4. Sprinkle dried dill, salt, and pepper.
5. Drizzle with olive oil.
6. Bake for 12-15 minutes or until the salmon is cooked through.
7. Meanwhile, toss the assorted vegetables with garlic powder, olive oil, salt, and pepper.
8. Spread the vegetables on a separate baking sheet and roast for 15-20 minutes or until tender.
9. Serve the baked salmon with roasted vegetables.

Day 22:

Meal 1 (Breakfast):
- Greek Yogurt with Berries and Almonds
Ingredients:
- 1 cup Greek yogurt
- Mixed berries (e.g., blueberries, strawberries, raspberries)
- Almonds, sliced
- Honey (optional)

Preparation:

1. In a bowl, scoop the Greek yogurt.

2. Top with mixed berries and sliced almonds.

3. Drizzle with honey if desired.

4. Enjoy!

Meal 2 (Lunch):

- Chicken Caesar Salad Wrap

Ingredients:

- Grilled chicken breast, sliced

- Romaine lettuce, chopped

- Cherry tomatoes, halved

- Parmesan cheese, grated

- Whole wheat tortilla

- Caesar dressing (look for a low-fat or homemade version)

Preparation:

1. Lay the whole wheat tortilla flat.

2. Spread Caesar dressing on the tortilla.

3. Layer romaine lettuce, sliced grilled chicken breast, cherry tomatoes, and grated Parmesan cheese.

4. Roll the tortilla into a wrap.

5. Serve fresh or lightly toasted.

Meal 3 (Dinner):

- Baked Chicken Thighs with Quinoa and Steamed Broccoli

Ingredients:

- 2 chicken thighs

- Lemon juice
- Garlic powder, paprika, and dried herbs for seasoning
- Olive oil
- Salt and pepper to taste
- 1/2 cup cooked quinoa
- Broccoli florets

Preparation:

1. Preheat the oven to 425°F (220°C).

2. Season the chicken thighs with lemon juice, garlic powder, paprika, dried herbs, salt, and pepper.

3. Drizzle with olive oil.

4. On a parchment paper-lined baking sheet, put the chicken thighs.

5. Bake for 25-30 minutes or until the chicken is cooked through and the skin is crispy.

6. Meanwhile, steam the broccoli florets until tender.

7. Serve the baked chicken thighs with cooked quinoa and steamed broccoli.

Day 23:

Meal 1 (Breakfast):
- **Spinach and Mushroom Omelette**
Ingredients:
- 2 eggs
- Spinach leaves
- Mushrooms, sliced
- Onion, diced

- Salt and pepper to taste
- Chopped fresh herbs (such as parsley or thyme).

Preparation:

1. Whisk the eggs with salt and pepper in a bowl
2. Heat a non-stick pan and sauté the mushrooms and onion until softened.
3. Once added, boil the spinach until it has wilted.
4. Pour the whisked eggs into the pan and cook until set.
5. Sprinkle fresh herbs on one side of the omelet.
6. Fold the omelet in half to cover the herbs.
7. Cook for another minute.
8. Slice and serve.

Meal 2 (Lunch):

- Mediterranean Quinoa Salad

Ingredients:

- 1/2 cup cooked quinoa
- Cucumber, diced
- Cherry tomatoes, halved
- Red onion, thinly sliced
- Kalamata olives
- Feta cheese, crumbled
- Fresh parsley, chopped
- Lemon juice and olive oil dressing
- Salt and pepper to taste

Preparation:

1. In a bowl, combine the cooked quinoa, cucumber, cherry tomatoes, red onion, Kalamata olives, feta cheese, and fresh parsley.

2. Drizzle with lemon juice and olive oil dressing.

3. Season with salt and pepper.

4. Toss gently to mix well.

Meal 3 (Dinner):

- Baked Cod with Quinoa and Steamed Asparagus

Ingredients:

- 4 oz cod filet

- Lemon juice

- Dried herbs (such as Rosemary or thyme)

- Olive oil

- Salt and pepper to taste

- 1/2 cup cooked quinoa

- Asparagus spears

Preparation:

1. Preheat the oven to 400°F (200°C).

2. On a baking sheet covered with parchment paper, put the cod filet.

3. Squeeze lemon juice over the fish.

4. Sprinkle dried herbs, salt, and pepper.

5. Drizzle with olive oil.

6. Bake for 12-15 minutes or until the fish is cooked through.

7. Meanwhile, steam the asparagus spears until tender.

8. Serve the baked cod with cooked quinoa and steamed asparagus.

Day 24:

Meal 1 (Breakfast):
- Berry Protein Smoothie
Ingredients:
- 1 cup unsweetened almond milk
- 1 scoop of the protein powder you choose
- Mixed berries (e.g., strawberries, blueberries, raspberries)
- 1 tbsp almond butter
- Ice cubes (optional)
Preparation:
1. In a blender, combine the almond milk, protein powder, mixed berries, almond butter, and ice cubes.
2. Blend until smooth and creamy.
3. Pour into a glass and enjoy.

Meal 2 (Lunch):
- Greek Salad with Grilled Chicken
Ingredients:
- Grilled chicken breast, sliced
- Mixed salad greens
- Cucumber, sliced
- Cherry tomatoes, halved
- Red onion, thinly sliced

- Kalamata olives
- Feta cheese, crumbled
- Lemon juice and olive oil dressing
- Dried oregano

Preparation:

1. Toss the salad greens, cucumber, cherry tomatoes, red onion, Kalamata olives, and feta cheese in a bowl.
2. Add the sliced grilled chicken on top.
3. Drizzle with lemon juice and olive oil dressing.
4. Sprinkle dried oregano.
5. Toss gently to mix well.

Meal 3 (Dinner):
- Grilled Steak with Roasted Vegetables
Ingredients:
- 4 oz steak (such as sirloin or ribeye)
- Salt and pepper to taste
- Olive oil
- Assorted vegetables (e.g., bell peppers, zucchini, eggplant)
- Garlic powder
- Olive oil
- Salt and pepper to taste

Preparation:

1. Preheat the grill.
2. Season the steak with salt and pepper.
3. Drizzle with olive oil.
4. Grill the steak to your desired level of doneness.

5. Meanwhile, toss the assorted vegetables with garlic powder, olive oil, salt, and pepper.

6. Spread the vegetables on a separate baking sheet and roast for 15-20 minutes or until tender.

7. Before slicing, let the steak rest for a few minutes.

8. Serve the grilled steak with roasted vegetables.

Day 25:

Meal 1 (Breakfast):
- Veggie Scramble
Ingredients:
- 2 eggs
- Bell peppers, diced
- Onion, diced
- Spinach leaves
- Tomatoes, diced
- Salt and pepper to taste
-Chopped fresh herbs (such as basil or parsley).
Preparation:
1. Whisk the eggs with salt and pepper in a bowl

2. Heat a non-stick pan and sauté the bell peppers and onion until softened.

3. Once added, boil the spinach until it has wilted.

4. Add the tomatoes and fresh herbs, and cook for another minute.

5. Pour the whisked eggs into the pan and scramble until cooked.

6. Serve hot.

Meal 2 (Lunch):
- Lentil Soup with Side Salad
Ingredients:
- 1 cup cooked lentils
- Carrot, diced
- Celery, diced
- Onion, diced
- Garlic, minced
- Vegetable broth
- Cumin, paprika, and dried herbs for seasoning
- Salt and pepper to taste
- Mixed salad greens
- Cherry tomatoes, halved
- Cucumber, sliced
- Balsamic vinegar and olive oil dressing

Preparation:
1. In a pot, sauté the carrot, celery, onion, and garlic until softened.
2. Add the cooked lentils and vegetable broth.
3. Season with cumin, paprika, dried herbs, salt, and pepper.
4. Simmer for 15-20 minutes.
5. Adjust the seasoning if needed.
6. Serve the lentil soup with a side salad of mixed greens, cherry tomatoes, and cucumber.
7. Drizzle with balsamic vinegar and olive oil dressing.

Meal 3 (Dinner):
- Baked Chicken Breast with Steamed Broccoli
Ingredients:
- 4 oz chicken breast
- Lemon juice
- Garlic powder, paprika, and dried herbs for seasoning
- Olive oil
- Salt and pepper to taste
- Broccoli florets
Preparation:
1. Preheat the oven to 400°F (200°C).
2. Season the chicken breast with lemon juice, garlic powder, paprika, dried herbs, salt, and pepper.
3. Drizzle with olive oil.
4. Place the chicken breast on a baking sheet lined with parchment paper.
5. Bake the chicken for 20 to 25 minutes, or until cooked through.
6. Meanwhile, steam the broccoli florets until tender.
7. Serve the baked chicken breast with steamed broccoli.

Day 26:

Meal 1 (Breakfast):
- Avocado Toast with Poached Eggs
Ingredients:
- Whole wheat bread (toasted)

- Ripe avocado, mashed
- Poached eggs
- Salt and pepper to taste
- Red pepper flakes (optional)

Preparation:

1. Toast the whole wheat bread.

2. Spread mashed avocado on the toast.

3. Place a poached egg on top of the avocado.

4. Season with salt, pepper, and red pepper flakes if desired.

5. Enjoy!

Meal 2 (Lunch):

- Quinoa Salad with Roasted Vegetables

Ingredients:

- 1/2 cup cooked quinoa
- Assorted roasted vegetables (e.g., sweet potatoes, Brussels sprouts, bell peppers)
- Spinach leaves
- Cherry tomatoes, halved
- Red onion, thinly sliced
- Feta cheese, crumbled
- Lemon juice and olive oil dressing
- Salt and pepper to taste

Preparation:

1. In a bowl, combine the cooked quinoa, roasted vegetables, spinach leaves, cherry tomatoes, red onion, and feta cheese.

2. Drizzle with lemon juice and olive oil dressing.

3. Season with salt and pepper.

4. Toss gently to mix well.

Meal 3 (Dinner):
- Salmon baked with quinoa and asparagus steaming
Ingredients:
- 4 oz salmon filet
- Lemon juice
- Dried dill
- Olive oil
- Salt and pepper to taste
- 1/2 cup cooked quinoa
- Asparagus spears

Preparation:
1. Preheat the oven to 400°F (200°C).

2. Place the salmon filet on a baking sheet lined with parchment paper.

3. Squeeze lemon juice over the fish.

4. Sprinkle dried dill, salt, and pepper.

5. Drizzle with olive oil.

6. Bake for 12-15 minutes or until the fish is cooked through.

7. Meanwhile, steam the asparagus spears until tender.

8. Serve the baked salmon with cooked quinoa and steamed asparagus.

Day 27:

Meal 1 (Breakfast):
- Veggie Breakfast Burrito
Ingredients:
- Whole wheat tortilla
- Scrambled eggs
- Bell peppers, diced
- Onion, diced
- Spinach leaves
- Shredded cheese (such as cheddar or mozzarella)
- Salsa or hot sauce (optional)
Preparation:
1. Lay the whole wheat tortilla flat.
2. Spread scrambled eggs on the tortilla.
3. Layer diced bell peppers, diced onion, spinach leaves, and shredded cheese.
4. Add salsa or hot sauce if desired.
5. Roll the tortilla into a burrito.
6. Serve fresh or lightly toasted.

Meal 2 (Lunch):
- Chickpea and Vegetable Stir-Fry
Ingredients:
- 1 cup cooked chickpeas
- Assorted stir-fry vegetables (e.g., bell peppers, broccoli, snap peas, carrots)
- Garlic, minced

- Soy sauce or tamari
- Sesame oil
- Salt and pepper to taste
- Cooked brown rice or quinoa (optional)

Preparation:

1. Heat a pan with a little sesame oil.
2. Sauté the minced garlic until fragrant.
3. Add the stir-fry vegetables and cooked chickpeas.
4. Cook until the vegetables are tender-crisp.
5. Drizzle with soy sauce or tamari and toss to coat.
6. Season with salt and pepper.
7. Serve the chickpea and vegetable stir-fry as is or with cooked brown rice or quinoa.

Meal 3 (Dinner):
- Grilled Chicken with Greek Salad
Ingredients:

- Grilled chicken breast, sliced
- Mixed salad greens
- Cucumber, sliced
- Cherry tomatoes, halved
- Red onion, thinly sliced
- Kalamata olives
- Feta cheese, crumbled
- Lemon juice and olive oil dressing
- Dried oregano

Preparation:

1. Toss the salad greens, cucumber, cherry tomatoes, red onion, Kalamata olives, and feta cheese in a bowl.
2. Add the sliced grilled chicken on top.
3. Drizzle with lemon juice and olive oil dressing.
4. Sprinkle dried oregano.
5. Toss gently to mix well.

Day 28:

Meal 1 (Breakfast):
- Spinach and Mushroom Frittata
Ingredients:
- 2 eggs
- Spinach leaves
- Mushrooms, sliced
- Onion, diced
- Salt and pepper to taste
- Chopped fresh herbs (such as thyme or parsley).
Preparation:
1. Whisk the eggs with salt and pepper in a bowl
2. Heat a non-stick pan and sauté the mushrooms and onion until softened.
3. Once added, boil the spinach until it has wilted.
4. Pour the whisked eggs into the pan and cook until set.
5. Sprinkle fresh herbs on top.
6. Cook for another minute.
7. Slice and serve.

Meal 2 (Lunch):
- Greek Chicken Pita
Ingredients:
- Grilled chicken breast, sliced
- Whole wheat pita bread
- Tzatziki sauce (look for a low-fat or homemade version)
- Mixed salad greens
- Cucumber, sliced
- Cherry tomatoes, halved
- Red onion, thinly sliced
- Kalamata olives
- Feta cheese, crumbled
Preparation:
1. Open the whole wheat pita bread to form a pocket.
2. Spread tzatziki sauce inside the pocket.
3. Layer mixed salad greens, sliced grilled chicken breast, cucumber slices, cherry tomatoes, red onion, Kalamata olives, and crumbled feta cheese.
4. Serve fresh or lightly toasted.

Meal 3 (Dinner):
- Baked Cod with Quinoa and Steamed Broccoli
Ingredients:
- 4 oz cod filet
- Lemon juice
- Dried herbs (such as Rosemary or thyme)
- Olive oil

- Salt and pepper to taste
- 1/2 cup cooked quinoa
- Broccoli florets

Preparation:
1. Preheat the oven to 400°F (200°C).
2. On a baking sheet covered with parchment paper, put the fish filet.
3. Squeeze lemon juice over the fish.
4. Sprinkle dried herbs, salt, and pepper.
5. Drizzle with olive oil.
6. Bake for 12-15 minutes or until the fish is cooked through.
7. Meanwhile, steam the broccoli florets until tender.
8. Serve the baked cod with cooked quinoa and steamed broccoli.

Day 29:

Meal 1 (Breakfast):
- **Berry and Spinach Smoothie**
Ingredients:
- 1 cup almond milk (unsweetened)
- Mixed berries (e.g., blueberries, strawberries, raspberries)
- Spinach leaves
- 1 tbsp almond butter
- Ice cubes (optional)

Preparation:

1. In a blender, combine the almond milk, mixed berries, spinach leaves, almond butter, and ice cubes.

2. Blend until smooth and creamy.

3. Pour into a glass and enjoy.

Meal 2 (Lunch):
- Greek Salad Wrap
Ingredients:
- Whole wheat tortilla
- Mixed salad greens
- Cucumber, sliced
- Cherry tomatoes, halved
- Red onion, thinly sliced
- Kalamata olives
- Feta cheese, crumbled
- Lemon juice and olive oil dressing
- Dried oregano

Preparation:

1. Lay the whole wheat tortilla flat.

2. Spread mixed salad greens on the tortilla.

3. Layer cucumber slices, cherry tomatoes, red onion, Kalamata olives, and crumbled feta cheese.

4. Drizzle with lemon juice and olive oil dressing.

5. Sprinkle dried oregano.

6. Roll the tortilla into a wrap.

7. Serve fresh or lightly toasted.

Meal 3 (Dinner):
- Baked Chicken Thighs with Roasted Vegetables
Ingredients:
- 2 chicken thighs
- Lemon juice
- Garlic powder, paprika, and dried herbs for seasoning
- Olive oil
- Salt and pepper to taste
- Assorted vegetables (e.g., bell peppers, zucchini, eggplant)
- Garlic powder
- Olive oil
- Salt and pepper to taste

Preparation:
1. Preheat the oven to 425°F (220°C).
2. Season the chicken thighs with lemon juice, garlic powder, paprika, dried herbs, salt, and pepper.
3. Drizzle with olive oil.
4. On a parchment paper-lined baking sheet, put the chicken thighs.
5. Bake for 25-30 minutes or until the chicken is cooked through and the skin is crispy.
6. Meanwhile, toss the assorted vegetables with garlic powder, olive oil, salt, and pepper.
7. Spread the vegetables on a separate baking sheet and roast for 15-20 minutes or until tender.
8. Serve the baked chicken thighs with roasted vegetables.

Day 30:

Meal 1 (Breakfast):
- **Veggie Omelette**
Ingredients:
- 2 eggs
- Bell peppers, diced
- Onion, diced
- Spinach leaves
- Tomatoes, diced
- Salt and pepper to taste
- Chopped fresh herbs (such as parsley or basil).
Preparation:
1. Whisk the eggs with salt and pepper in a bowl
2. Heat a non-stick pan and sauté the bell peppers and onion until softened.
3. Once added, boil the spinach until it has wilted.
4. Add the tomatoes and fresh herbs, and cook for another minute.
5. Pour the whisked eggs into the pan and cook until set.
6. Fold the omelet in half and cook for an additional minute.
7. Slice and serve.

Meal 2 (Lunch):
- **Mediterranean Quinoa Bowl**
Ingredients:
- 1/2 cup cooked quinoa

- Cucumber, diced
- Cherry tomatoes, halved
- Red onion, thinly sliced
- Kalamata olives
- Feta cheese, crumbled
- Fresh parsley, chopped
- Lemon juice
- Olive oil
- Salt and pepper to taste

Preparation:

1. In a bowl, combine the cooked quinoa, cucumber, cherry tomatoes, red onion, Kalamata olives, feta cheese, and fresh parsley.
2. Squeeze lemon juice over the quinoa bowl.
3. Drizzle with olive oil.
4. Season with salt and pepper.
5. Toss gently to mix well.

Meal 3 (Dinner):
- **Baked Salmon with Steamed Broccoli**
Ingredients:
- 4 oz salmon filet
- Lemon juice
- Dried dill
- Olive oil
- Salt and pepper to taste
- Broccoli florets

Preparation:

1. Preheat the oven to 400°F (200°C).
2. Place the salmon filet on a baking sheet lined with parchment paper.
3. Squeeze lemon juice over the fish.
4. Sprinkle dried dill, salt, and pepper.
5. Drizzle with olive oil.
6. Bake for 12-15 minutes or until the fish is cooked through.
7. Meanwhile, steam the broccoli florets until tender.
8. Serve the baked salmon with steamed broccoli.

Remember to adjust portion sizes and ingredient quantities based on your individual needs. Enjoy your meals!

CONCLUSION

In conclusion, **"INTERMITTENT FASTING FOR WOMEN OVER 50"** is a comprehensive and informative guide that empowers women in this age group to embrace intermittent fasting as a beneficial and sustainable lifestyle choice. The book has explored the unique considerations and potential benefits of intermittent fasting for women over 50, providing valuable insights and practical strategies for success.

Throughout the book, the authors have addressed the specific physiological changes that occur with age, offering tailored guidance on how to adapt the fasting approach to suit the needs of women in this demographic. From hormonal fluctuations to metabolic changes, the book provides a clear understanding of how intermittent fasting can positively impact various aspects of health and well-being.

The authors have also emphasized the importance of personalized approaches and the need for individual experimentation and adjustment. By encouraging readers to consult with healthcare professionals, monitor their progress, and listen to their bodies, the book promotes a safe and sustainable journey into intermittent fasting.

One of the book's strengths is its wealth of practical tools and resources. It includes sample meal plans, fasting schedules, and a diverse range of delicious recipes that cater to the nutritional needs of women over 50. The authors have thoughtfully considered the importance of nutrient density, incorporating key vitamins, minerals, and macronutrients into the suggested meal options.

Overall, **"INTERMITTENT FASTING FOR WOMEN OVER 50"** serves as a comprehensive and empowering guide that equips women in this age group with the knowledge, tools, and confidence to embrace intermittent fasting as a transformative lifestyle practice. It provides valuable insights, practical strategies, and inspiring success stories, making it an invaluable resource for any woman seeking to improve her health, vitality, and overall well-being.